I'll Love You Forever

Jody Guler

Bloomington, IN 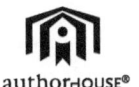 Milton Keynes, UK

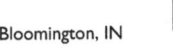

AuthorHouse™
1663 Liberty Drive, Suite 200
Bloomington, IN 47403
www.authorhouse.com
Phone: 1-800-839-8640

AuthorHouse™ UK Ltd.
500 Avebury Boulevard
Central Milton Keynes, MK9 2BE
www.authorhouse.co.uk
Phone: 08001974150

Cover photo: December 1988 (family photo)

First published by AuthorHouse   1/12/2007

ISBN: 978-1-4259-8056-6 (sc)

Library of Congress Control Number: 2006911027

Printed in the United States of America
Bloomington, Indiana

This book is printed on acid-free paper.

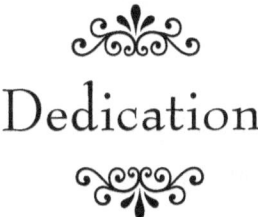

Dedication

To my parents, Thomas and Geraldine Strong: Thank you for giving me life, teaching me how to love, and for creating such a wonderful family and home. Your love and devotion to each other always made me feel very secure. I am proud to be your daughter.

To my husband Dan, whom I have loved since I was sixteen years old: Thank you for your unconditional love, for always treating me like a queen, and for sharing your life with me. I pray our daughters are blessed with a husband as amazing and devoted as you. My love for you is unending.

For my daughters Meghan and Allison: My love for both of you is unalterable, unexplainable, and undying. You have brought much joy and pleasure into my life. You will only realize how much I love you when you have children of your own.

To my brothers and sisters: I cherish and love each one of you and your families. God has richly blessed me with such supportive and loving siblings; thank you for your love.

Before I begin to tell you my story, I would like to share some things about my father with you. I want you to know more about him than just his life during his illness. He was a loving, soft-hearted, kind man who had a great sense of humor and treasured his family.

My father, Tom Strong, was born July 12, 1923 to Harry and Stella Strong in Osseo, Wisconsin. He was one of six children. Growing up, Dad lost his three brothers, all at young ages. His family went through many tragic losses and much unbearable pain. He had two remaining sisters whom he loved dearly.

At an early age, music became the focal point of his life. When he was four years old, being billed as "Professor Littleman," and dressed in a stovepipe hat and tails, he played his trumpet for an event at the high school. He experienced a little stage fright and literally had to be carried onto the stage. However, once he started playing his favorite song, "Among My Souvenirs," he wouldn't stop. Again he had to be carried, this time off of the stage.

Dad played basketball and lettered all four years in high school and then served as a pharmacist's mate in the U.S. Navy during WWII aboard a tanker ship, the U.S.S. Escambia.

After returning home, he met his future wife Geraldine Lightfoot (Jerry Lou), and they married February 3, 1951. This union of love brought six children, and eventually those children's spouses and grandchildren. Dad's family was his love and his life.

My father worked in the lumber business, and everyone who knew him professionally became his personal friend. He went out of his way to help his customers in any way that he could.

Dad continued to play his trumpet and enjoyed entertaining people with his love of music by playing in a dance band. His enthusiasm for music carried on to his children and grandchildren.

He retired at the age of sixty-five—just months prior to his diagnosis. Looking forward to retirement, he and my mother were going to enjoy time together after raising six children.

My father led us by example and taught us how to be good Christians through his actions and words.

Shortly after my father died, I wrote his story and gave it to my family members as a Christmas gift. I had been the first person who heard the words God had spoken to him, and therefore I felt it was my responsibility to put it down in writing so the exact words and facts would never be forgotten.

Over the years I have recounted my father's story with many people who have lost loved ones. It is something people hunger to hear. After thanking me for telling them, others have expressed to me how much peace and consolation it brought to them. They craved the reassurance that their loved ones were in a better place, and that they would see them again.

Now, years later, I feel it is my obligation to share what I wrote for my family with others. It is something so remarkable and miraculous that I feel it needs to be told.

Thank you for letting me share my father's story with you.

Jody Guler

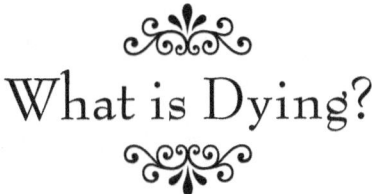

What is Dying?

The ship sails and I stand watching till she fades on the horizon, And someone at my side says, "She is gone." Gone where? Gone from my sight, that is all; she is just as large as when I saw her.

The diminished size and total loss of sight is in me, not in her, and just at that moment, when someone at my side says, "She Is gone." There are others who are watching her coming, and Other voices take up a glad shout. "There she comes!"

And that is dying.

Bishop Brent

This is a true story of the journey that I was part of after my father, Thomas Strong Sr., was diagnosed with cancer on January 19, 1989. For the following nine months, I watched this kind, loving, and wonderful husband, father, grandfather, and friend, go through months of agonizing pain, and then his passing. But through all of this, he remained a remarkable man, giving us strength when we needed it and always remaining faithful and loving to God. I had no idea what I was about to witness when I looked in on him in his room on the morning of May 18, 1989.

Please read his story and pass it on to a family member or friend so that you and others may also be given the strength to remain hopeful and faithful during a very difficult and painful time.

I promise you that you will see your loved one again; my father told me so...

"I'll Love You Forever"

The beautiful locket was wrapped in a lovely, small gift box. My mother tearfully waited to receive the gift from my father's weak but loving hand. It required several of us to help raise our father's arm so he could place this special gift into our mother's trembling hands. We all knew deep in our hearts that this would be the last Mother's Day gift that our father would ever give to her. The week before, my sisters and I tried to think of a meaningful present that Dad could give to our mother, and decided on this charming locket. Our father was growing weaker; the painful, degrading disease of cancer was slowly taking this wonderful, loving man away from us.

We were still desperately praying that God would perform a miracle and Dad would survive. We couldn't imagine our lives without him in them. He was always there for each of us and loved his family and grandchildren very much. We wanted our children to have their Grandfather whom they adored, in their lives. Men and fathers like Dad were role models, and we needed people like him on earth. God didn't need him in heaven; we needed him more here.

All twenty-two of us were crammed into the small den in my parent's home: my mother and father, two brothers, three sisters, spouses, my husband and I, and every grandchild. My father lay weak in the recliner that we had delivered to the house prior to his arrival home from the hospital after his biopsy. During the day, Dad spent many hours in this chair, in this room, and in this house. He slept, ate, watched television, took his medicine, listened to music (he was a wonderful musician who played the trumpet in a small dance band in the area), and when he had better days, he visited with friends and relatives who had stopped to see him. This is where he recuperated after each chemotherapy and radiation treatment. The person he spent most of his hours with in this room was my mother. He did not want to be in his bed during the day—that would have meant he was sick!

We watched, our eyes burning with tears, as mom looked at her gift. She couldn't imagine what this tiny box held. As she opened it, we all took turns gazing at her and Dad. He was so frail, so ill, and we loved them both so very much; we could hardly stand watching them when they were both in so much pain. Mom took her present out of the box. It was a beautiful locket on a delicate chain. She held it up for all to see. Someone told her to turn it over, and mom wept as she read the inscription. My sister who had selected the locket had tried to speak to my dad so that he could choose the words he would like engraved on the locket for mom. This took patience from her because Dad had not been very coherent during the week prior to

Mother's Day. She persisted because she wanted the words to come from our father. Eventually he was able to tell her, and speaking in his fragile voice, he said,

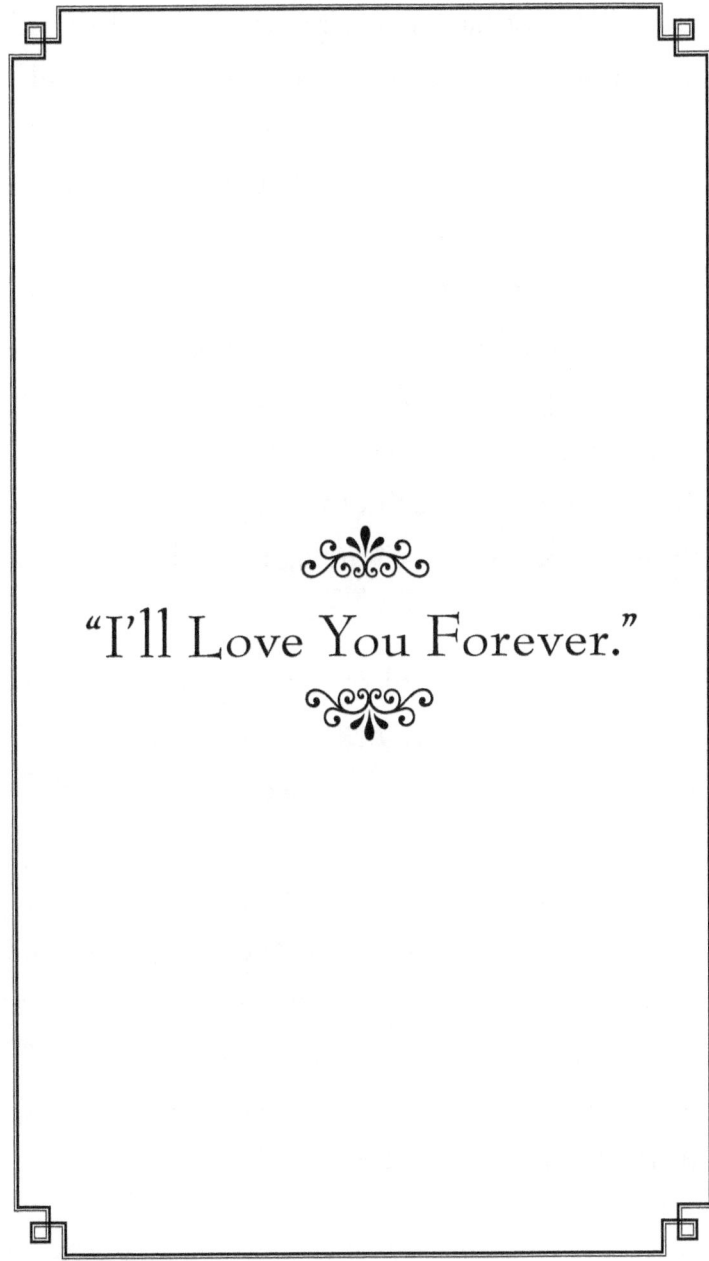

"I'll Love You Forever."

These were special, endearing words that they had shared with each other for the past thirty-eight years of married life. Growing up, I remember seeing those words on cards they shared with each other. It was something very dear and meaning-ful to both of them. My parents met in 1948 and were married in 1951. Their love for one another grew stronger with each passing year. These past four months had been difficult for both of them; they tried to keep each other's spirits up, though all the while they were hurting for each other very deeply.

Our mother leaned over my father who was lying feeble in his chair. Sobbing, she thanked him, embraced him, and cried. We all cried as they shared a painful, yet very tender, moment of their love for one another. There was never a time in our lives that we doubted their true love and respect for each other. They had a relationship that we all wanted to know in our marriages. It hurt us all to see them both suffering, each locked into a different kind of pain.

It was a Sunday afternoon, and five out of the six families had to return to their homes in different cities. All of us had made this trip many times since our father had been diagnosed with cancer in January. Dad had been a healthy man all of his life, and had only visited the doctor once in the thirty-eight years that my parents had been married. When my mother noticed him experiencing pain in his shoulder, she tried to get him to see the doctor to get something to help ease his discomfort. Dad didn't think it was necessary, and put it off. He'd chalk the pain up to different things, and would say things like, "I must have hurt it lifting something at work," or, "I must have hurt it when I was helping the guys lift an instrument into the van," or, "Maybe this is just bursitis." But by Christmas, it was obvious the pain in his shoulder was worse, and we were all nagging him to promise to see someone about it right after the holidays. He promised us he would.

When Dad finally let our mother schedule an appointment for him in January, we knew he couldn't cope with the suffering anymore. They were planning to celebrate their thirty-eighth wedding anniversary with a trip in February. They were going to drive to Alabama to visit my mother's relatives, retracing their original honeymoon. Dad agreed that he should get his shoulder examined and get something stronger for the pain before they left.

My parents went to the appointment together. Following his examination, the doctor told my father that he was going to give him something for his pain and inflammation. But just as the doctor was about to leave the room, he asked my father how long it had been since his last chest x-ray. My father, having gone to the doctor just the once in the past thirty-eight years and having been treated for bursitis, had no recollection of ever having had a chest x-ray. The doctor suggested my father have an x-ray taken for his medical records before he left. After the x-ray, my parents left the clinic assuming all Dad needed to do to help his condition improve was to take the prescriptions that the doctor had prescribed for him. Relieved, they went home.

The next day my father received a phone call from the doctor's office that would turn his life and our family upside down.

He was told the x-ray showed a spot on one of his lungs, and the nurse stated the doctor wanted him to come back in for further tests. My father immediately called my mother at work and told her about the phone call. Startled and shocked, she called the clinic and asked to speak to the doctor directly. Dad's doctor spoke to my mother and proceeded to tell her on the phone that it didn't look good, and that they would know more after the tests. We all received a devastating phone call from our very terrified mother. Mom didn't want our dad to know she had talked to the doctor and she wasn't holding up well. "We all need to pray, she said, pray hard."

That very week, my father was scheduled for tests. My brother-in-law, Mark, and I were free to make the trip to be with my parents; our family agreed someone should be with them for this appointment. I will never forget that day as long as I live!

After drinking a liquid in preparation for the MRI, my dad was led into a room by a technician. The three of us—my mother, Mark, and I—stood outside the room. On the wall was a small window into the x-ray department, where we could actually see my father lying on a table. Located on a wall directly across from us was a large screen. We could see pictures being taken by the MRI machine, and we were able to view the machine circling areas over the images on the screen. What did all this mean? I was feeling nauseated and scared. I felt weak, and feared that these circles meant something was terribly wrong. Of course, I had no knowledge of this high tech machine and its testing, but I was certain all the circles and markings meant something alarming. When finished, the technician proceeded to help my father off the table; he was then out of our sight for a short while. My mother, nervously pacing in the hall, caught a glimpse of him seated in one of the examination rooms, and he mouthed to her, "It's not good, it's not good." My mother, in tears, came over to Mark and me and told us what my dad had just said. What was wrong with my dad? What had the test shown? One of the x-ray technicians spoke to us, saying, "The doctor would like to talk to you now." I felt myself weaken again, and began feeling lightheaded, as if I was falling; I was going to faint! I just knew the doctor was going to tell us something awful— something horrible. As my brother-in-law Mark held me and kept me on my feet, I told him that I couldn't go in there, that I didn't want to hear it. Mark spoke to me softly and said I had to be strong for my mom and dad, but I was pulling back. I didn't want to hear what the doctor was going to tell us. Mark walked me into the room, and by then both my parents were crying, and I knew the doctor had just revealed something devastating to them both.

Though we were fearful of what the doctor was going to reveal to us, we were not prepared for what he was about to say. The doctor told us my father had cancer that had metastasized to five parts of his body, including three areas of his spine. I thought to myself, *How dare you make up something like this to tell people, my father only came in with shoulder pain!* I just wouldn't believe it! The doctor actually stated that it was possible that my dad had only three more months to live while standing right in front of him! I rejected this terrible news and said, "Don't worry Dad, you can fight this, we will all help you." The doctor looked directly at me and said, "This should be your father's choice." I hated this man! He had just given my father a death sentence, and acted like there wasn't any hope at all. In the next breath, he dared to tell us he would be gone for the weekend and that he would be turning my father's case over to another physician. There was a tumor in my father's lung and a biopsy would be required to determine what kind of cancer he had. What did this man think he was doing, telling my father that he was terminally ill and then having the nerve to tell us he was going away for a weekend with his family to ski? To have fun! He would be having fun with his family though he had just destroyed ours!

Dad was hospitalized for a biopsy, and the results confirmed what the doctor had told us. His prognosis was very poor; the cancer had already invaded his bones. Our father, on his own, decided to go through chemotherapy and radiation treatments. He was going to put up a fight. His treatments required many trips to the oncology department in the hospital, and Dad was always brave and strong. Each treatment took some time for him to recover from, but all in all, after numerous doctor visits and treatments, they didn't seem to be having any positive effects on the cancer. The treatments continued for weeks, then months, and Dad was becoming more debilitated and ill.

That special Mother's Day marked almost four months since dad's diagnosis. Four, long months, that had consisted of tests, treatments, medicine, pain, daily phone calls, visits from relatives, each family's taking turns with visits home, and my mother's constant, loving care for my father. The treatments took their toll on him him, but he stayed strong and determined. My father was growing weaker, losing his hair, and losing a lot of weight, yet he still tried to maintain a positive attitude for all of us. I'm afraid he suffered much more than we will ever know. There were times when he would just collapse with pain due to muscle spasms, and whoever was beside him when this happened would be asked to rub the area. Sometimes when he dozed, you could see his muscles twitching and jumping. Everyone rubbed and helped however they could; even the grandchildren knew what to do to try to help Grandpa feel better.

Mother's Day weekend was over, and one by one each family said goodbye to dad during the late afternoon. We all cried and didn't want to leave, fearing that we were perhaps seeing Dad for the last time. What if this was forever? What if we would never be able to see him again? How do you say goodbye to your father for what could possibly be the last time? I know that each family member continued to pray for a miracle, but he was getting weaker, and we were afraid that God was not going to answer our prayer. The doctors didn't think he would be with us much longer. My youngest brother, Jim, was staying until Wednesday of the next week to help mom care for Dad, and as I left, I worried about Jim. Would he be the one to be with them if something happened in the next few days? I was to relieve him on Wednesday, and I wondered if Dad would last that long.

I cried and slept in cycles as I did every Sunday night on the way home after spending the weekend at my parents'. We had a three-hour drive, and all the way home I was filled with the emotion and pain that had been bottled up inside me after trying to stay strong for my parents. On the way home we would always pass by a church that was just off the highway in a small town called Rosendale. The girls, Dan, and I always enjoyed reading the sayings on the church's large sign outside. I woke up just as we were passing the church and looked over to read it. It said, "Take my hand Eternal Father, Strong to Survive." This surely was a sign from God, as my father's name was Tom Strong. He was going to live. God was sending me a sign; I just knew it!

I returned home three days later to relieve my brother Jim on Wednesday, May 17. Jim left in the morning to go home to Minneapolis. "He cried so hard when he left," mom said, "It was so terribly hard for him to leave Dad." Dad was failing even more, and my mother shared with me what had transpired that morning. Jim had heard my dad crying in his room when he had woken up. He ran to see what was happening, and my dad, in a very frail, shaking voice, explained that he had dreamt that he was drowning, and that in his dream, several people were pulling him under and others were pulling him back. My brother comforted him, and settled him down. Discussing the dream that morning, my mother and I reflected on my father's past. He had lost three brothers while he was growing up: two to illnesses and one to a tragic accident. He had also lost his parents, one sister, and his father-in-law. We wondered if they could have been the ones pulling him under, and if our family here could have been the ones pulling him back?

That night my mother and I settled my father into bed, went through the routine of giving him his medications, and then surrounded him with pillows to ease the pressure on his bones while he was lying down.

I seriously feared that Dad would die while I was there, and I also worried about him suffering terribly in the end. How would we comfort him? What would we do? I couldn't bear to see him suffer like this, but I also didn't want him to go. Dad had just retired the past fall, and he was only going to turn sixty-six years old. He was so young, and had so many more things he wanted to do. There would be more weddings, more grandchildren, and so many more years to share with mom in their retirement. He just couldn't die; how would we survive without him?

It was Wednesday evening, and my mother's aunt and uncle had also been at my father's side the last three days. They had come to stay at the house during the day to be of support to my mother, but in the evenings they returned to a hotel in town. I doubt that my father knew they were there; he slept most of the time. They left for the evening and my mother and I retreated to bed.

May 18

The next morning I rose and peeked in on Dad. I watched for his chest to rise and fall to reassure myself that he was okay. My mother and I visited with her aunt and uncle, who had returned to the house. The phone rang, and I ran to answer it so the ringing would not disturb my father. On the line was my sister Jane who lived in town. She was checking with us to see how Dad's night had gone and how things were going that morning. I hung up after speaking with her and went in to see if the phone had wakened him.

I Couldn't Believe What I Was Seeing!

There was my father, sitting up, on the side of the bed where my mother always slept. He was facing me, and although he looked weak and frail, he was alert. Prior to this, he had been unable to get into or out of his bed on his own. He looked like he was going to get right up out of bed! I asked, dumbfounded, "Dad, what are you doing?" In shock, I questioned him, "How did you get from your side of the bed to moms?" He had been nestled in pillows that we had carefully placed around him. How had he found the strength to move them aside and manage to sit up on his own? I'll forever remember my father's words. After hearing my questions, my father looked up at me and said clearly,

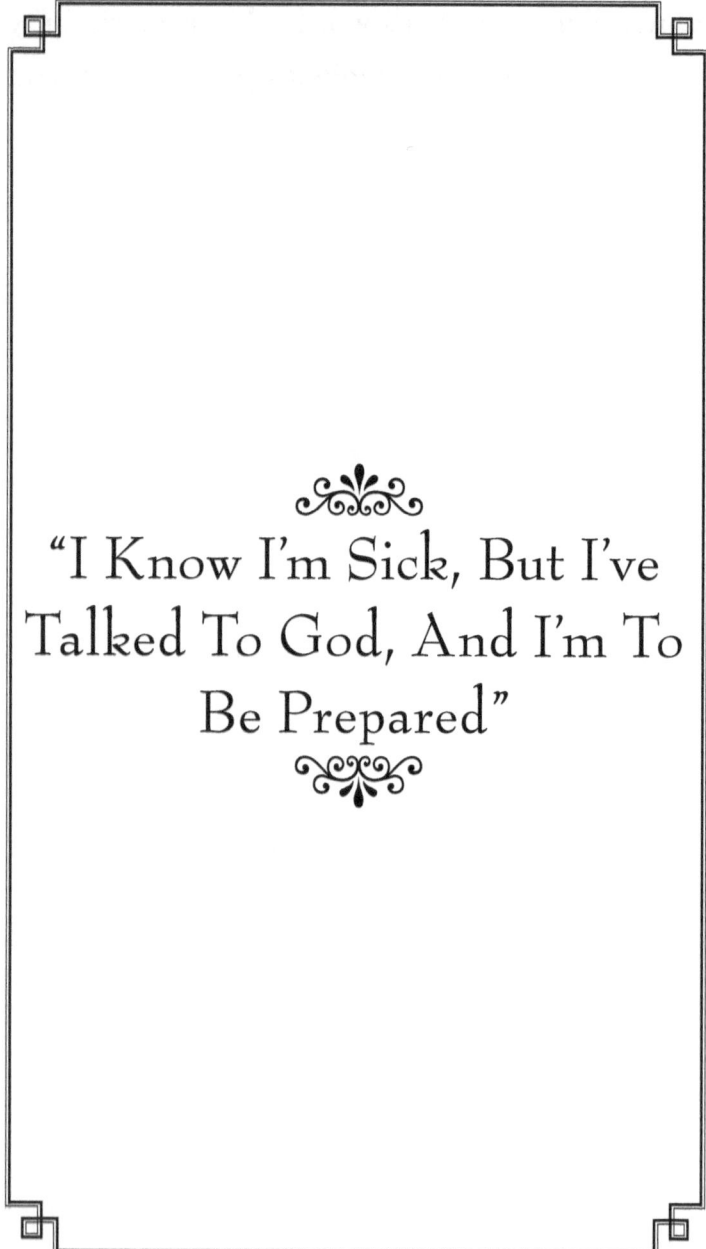

"I Know I'm Sick, But I've Talked To God, And I'm To Be Prepared"

I was already stunned that he was sitting up and talking clearly, and now my father was telling me that he had talked to God! All I could manage to say was, "Are you afraid?" Dad was still looking directly at me when he answered,

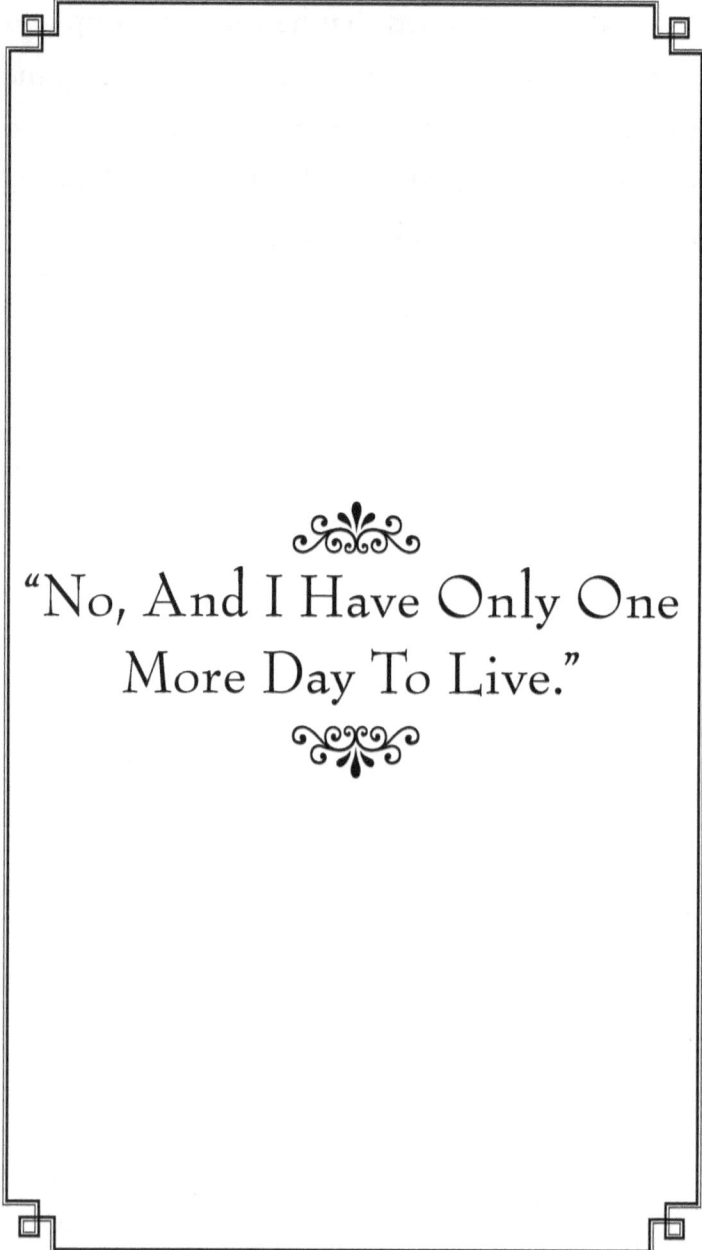

"No, And I Have Only One
More Day To Live."

I left him alone and ran crying into the living room to get my mother in order to bring her to their bedroom quickly. I told her that Dad was awake, alert, and sitting up, and I repeated to her what he had just said to me. My mother, not comprehending what I was telling her, swiftly returned with me to their bedroom. We found my dad beginning to get up out of bed on his own and telling us that he wanted to go into the living room. My mother was completely shocked. She, too, could not understand what was happening, but was overjoyed. Dad was mobile and talking clearly. Slowly, with one of us at each side, he walked into the living room and sat down in a chair. He proceeded to converse with Bob and Charlotte. They couldn't believe what they were witnessing either. (I later learned that they called home to their three children and families and told them that they had witnessed a miracle.)

As we sat together, Dad continued to speak to all of us as clearly as could be about most things. He told us he understood that he was ill, but that he did not remember any of the chemotherapy or radiation treatments we had told him about receiving. We listened to him, each amazed at what we were seeing and hearing. He did not recall the many weekly trips to the doctors, the tests, his treatments, or the family and friend visits with him and my mother. These traumatic and important events were completely erased from his mind. How could he not remember any of this? These past months of his life had been filled with all of these occurrences.

Grabbing the phone, I called my sister Jane. I told her to come quickly because Dad was up, alert, and moving around. I then made a phone call to his doctor's office and asked to speak immediately to his doctor. He took my call, and I explained to him what had just happened. Dad's physician said that he had seen many cases in which he believed people knew when their own deaths were coming, but he couldn't explain how our father, in his condition, could be up walking and speaking clearly with us. He told me he truthfully thought my father would not last through this week. He was amazed.

I next asked my mother if I should call our priest. She told me to call Father Krogman and tell him to come as soon as possible. Reaching Father Krogman, I explained what had taken place just minutes before, and related to him what Dad had told me when I walked into his room. Trying to talk through my tears, I told Father Krogman what my dad had said when I had found him sitting up in his bed. Repeating my father's words again, I told Father Krogman that he had looked up at me and plainly said,

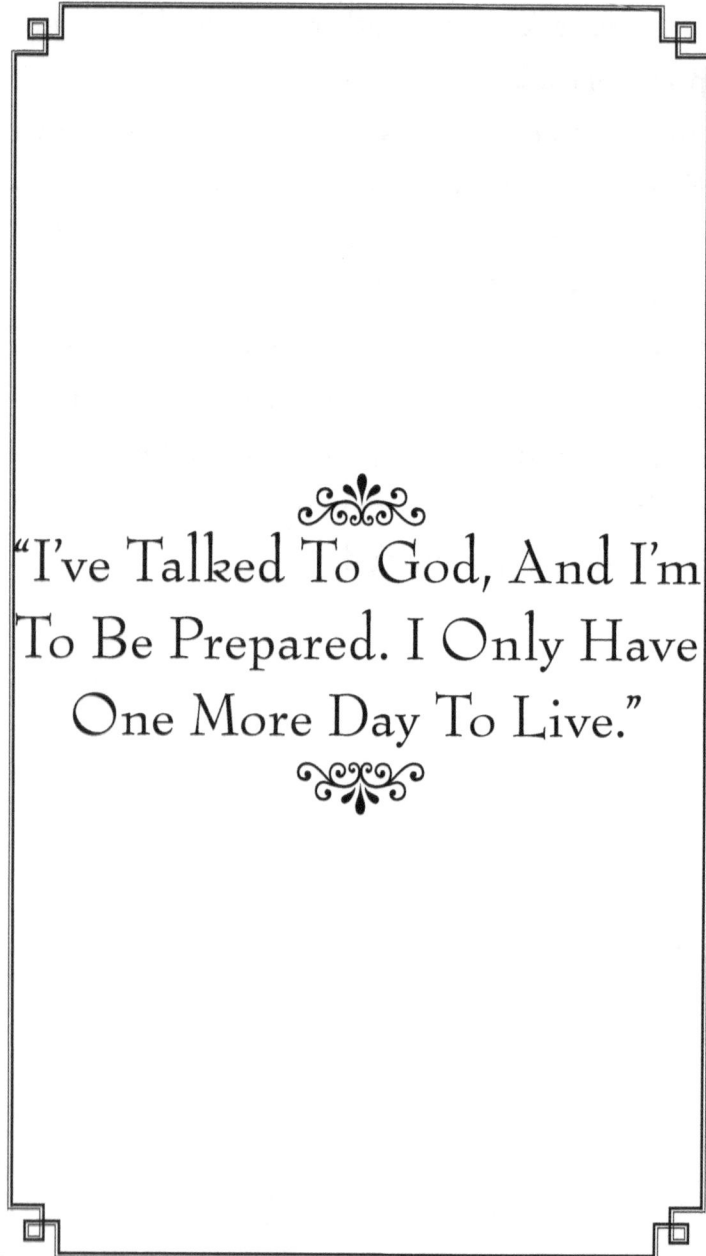

"I've Talked To God, And I'm
To Be Prepared. I Only Have
One More Day To Live."

Father Krogman promptly rushed over. He came into my parents' living room, spoke with my father, and then asked my sister, mother, and I to join him and my father in the den. Father Krogman had prayed and visited with my father and mother many times in this room. There we were—my mother, my sister, and I—surrounding Dad as we watched Father Krogman giving my father the sacrament of the last rites. I was very confused. I thought this was the miracle we had prayed for; my father was alert, his pain was not so excruciating, but he was also telling us he had only one more day to live. It was so surreal to be there witnessing my father receiving his blessing while all of us received Holy Communion together. What was happening? Did my father have only one more day to live, or were we all witnessing God performing a miracle that would allow him to survive?

As Father Krogman prayed over Dad, I prayed continuously and begged God for this to be the miracle we had all asked for: that our dad was to be healed and that he would live.

As I looked over at my dear father, with tears streaming down his face, he lifted his head up to heaven and asked out loud,

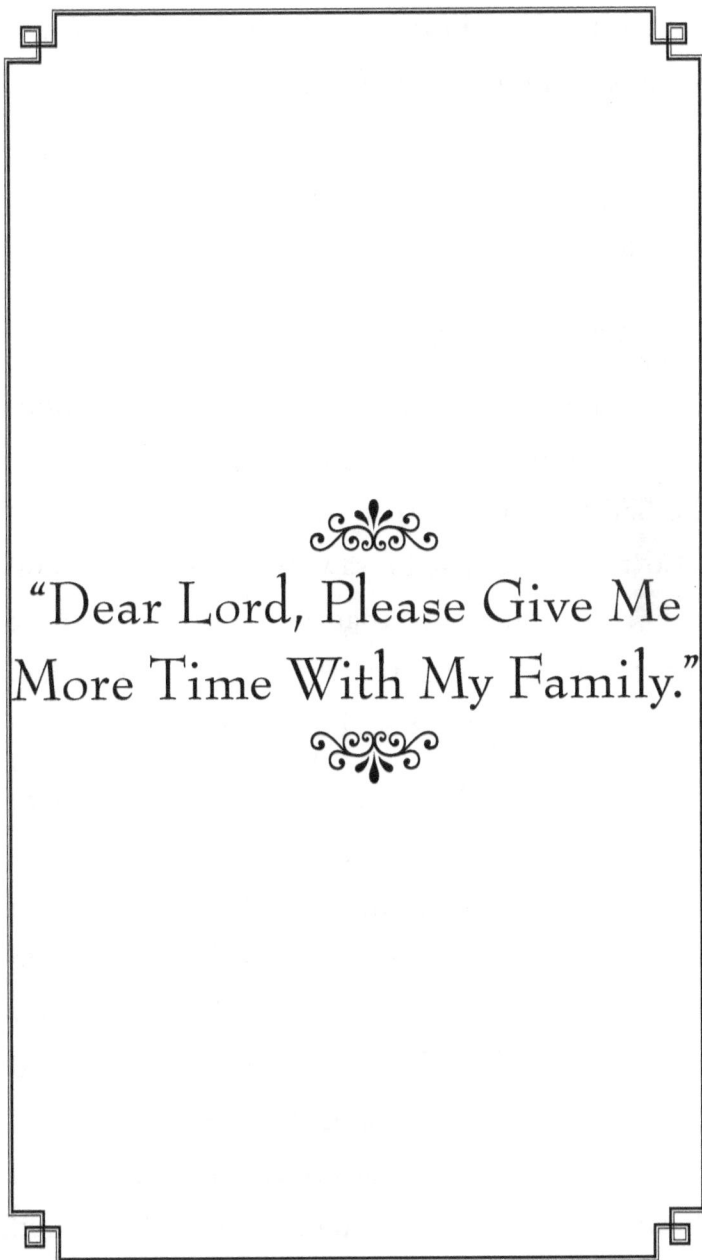

"Dear Lord, Please Give Me More Time With My Family."

I selfishly thought to myself, *no, Dad, ask God to cure you and to let you live.*

Father Krogman stayed with us for a while, and then left us to be together. Dad continued to get stronger throughout the day and evening.

It was a miracle.

During the day, Dad told my sister Jane about his dream of drowning. He repeated to her what he had told my brother Jim that morning. Dad also told Jane that he saw people he loved and missed so much, but that on the other hand, he wanted to stay with us. That night, he told her, God was going to make his decision.

That special day, May 18, was also my niece Rachel's birthday. A tradition of my parents was to call each of their children and grandchildren on his or her birthday, speak to him or her on two different phones, and sing "Happy Birthday To You" together. My mother and father called Rachel and began to sing. Dad, with his weak voice—though it was stronger now than it had been recently—was singing to his granddaughter.

I can't even imagine what they were thinking on the other end of the line at my brother's house. When they drove away on Mother's Day just four days earlier, I'm sure they thought the next phone call would be to tell them that Dad was gone. Instead, he was singing to Rachel! After speaking to Rachel, Dad spoke to my sister Jane and said to her, "Today [May 18] could be a dual occasion. It is Rachel Leigh Strong's birthday, and it could also be the day God calls me home."

After that phone call, my dad wanted to call his sister Annabelle, his only remaining sibling. Dad wanted to tell her that he loved her, and to thank her for coming to see him while he was sick, even though he did not recall her visits. He had learned that she had come to visit him along with her son Tom several times during the past months. I listened as he talked to his sister, and I heard him say,

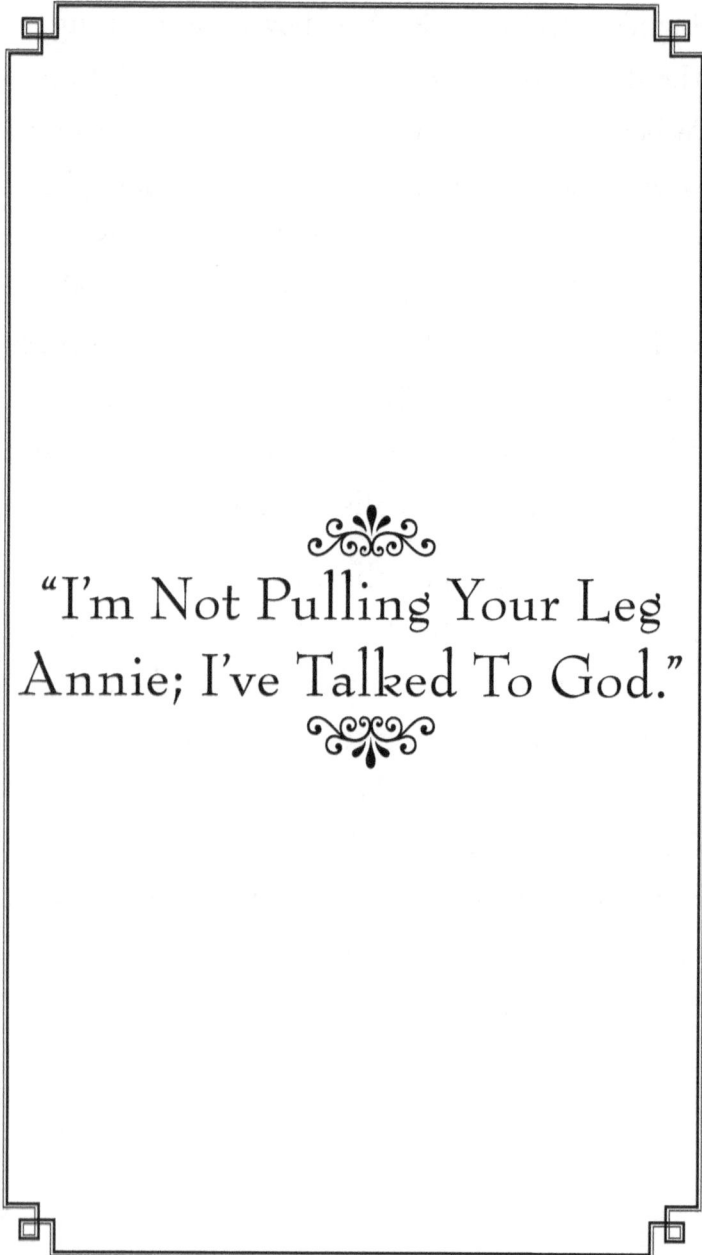

"I'm Not Pulling Your Leg Annie; I've Talked To God."

We called all of my brothers and sisters and told them what had taken place. They were all astonished and amazed. Dad asked the entire family to come home so he could see them again and talk to them. Overjoyed, everyone returned home. We were all gathered together once more in my parents home.

A few times when Dad heard someone arriving, he got up and hid behind the front door to surprise them as they came in. They couldn't believe what they were seeing! Dad had told us he had one more day to live, but he was up on his own and feeling stronger. It was an unbelievable turn, but what did all this mean? Everyone was very elated, yet very confused and unsure as to how to feel. We were all witnessing a miracle; our father seemed to be getting better, but yet he had told us he had only one more day to live.

Everyone stayed and we talked late into the evening of the day's events. Some of the family helped settle Dad into bed that evening. I remember him being very restless and not being able to relax and go to sleep. Sleep had been coming easily for him these past months, and that evening he fought it. He had prayed to God for more time with his family. Was God going to answer his prayer, or was he going to be called home?

The next morning, my father woke, and continued to be alert and strong. He told us that if this was to be his last day with us, there was something he needed to do. My father asked to speak privately with each of his children—both those who were married with their families and spouses, as well as the single ones—alone with him and my mother.

I'll forever remember my mother sitting on the sofa in the den reaching over and holding my father's hand while he was in his chair, and the love that was pouring out of my father's heart and soul. He told me many times how very much he loved me and how proud he was of me. Dad said he didn't want to die, but that he had been given a wonderful life. He told my husband Dan that he was very proud of him and loved him like a son. We had recently moved to Neenah, Wisconsin to start his new chiropractic practice.

My father told him that it took "a lot of guts" to sell an established practice in your hometown and move to a city where you knew no one, and to work so very hard. Dad asked his granddaughters, Meghan, who was then ten, and Allison, who was seven, if they were ever going to play a musical instrument. Music was a big part of his life, and he enjoyed playing his trumpet for anyone, especially his grandchildren. He told them that he loved them very much. Though we were receiving a blessing and gift from God and my father, it was very emotionally difficult to go through.

My father had some words to share with us that he felt were very important. *He told us that he would pass on the good word about us when he got to heaven, and that he would be there waiting. He said that he would save a spot for each of us, and that we should never, ever be afraid to die. He assured us it would be beautiful and wonderful, and that he would be waiting there for each of us when our time came.*

My brothers, sisters, and I all remember my father asking these three things of us:

To love one another
Not to fight with one another and
To take care of our mother

My sister Kim shared these words that Dad had said to her and her family: "Don't ever be afraid, it's such an easy feeling, that anyone could have taken me away. But I asked God for more time with my family; I wasn't ready to go."

God Heard His Prayer

May 19 passed, and so did several more months. God had listened to my father's prayer, and granted him more time with us.

Still very ill, but able to be more mobile, my father spent the next months making visits with my mother to each of our homes. One sister lived in Cuba City; the other five lived in different cities. My mother would prop my father's fragile and thin body with pillows in the front seat of the car. Carrying morphine in a bag between them, off they would go to visit one of their childrens' families. Dad was in intense pain again from the disease of cancer, but he was determined to see each of us in our own home and environment once more.

We were in the process of buying and redecorating an older home that we would be moving into and dad wanted to see it. It was two stories tall, and he was determined to climb the stairs and see the second floor. He was terribly feeble, but he made it. Our mother was wonderful; she helped him obtain his goal of visiting each family by traveling when Dad was a little stronger, then returning home so he could rest, then setting out again once more, and continuing this cycle until they had been to all of our homes. It wasn't easy for them, but Dad was determined to make these trips.

Also during this time, he would go to church and pray with my mom or sister, and make trips to Sinsinawa, the Dominican motherhouse that was near our home. He prayed many times with the nuns, and visited the chapel there. Several of the nuns made numerous trips to our parents' home when Dad couldn't travel, and they prayed there with him and my mother.

My sister Jane told me of a time she and Dad went together to pray. Jane had gone through a very painful divorce, and Mom and Dad were always there for her and her young daughter. "We were sitting in the pew," Jane said, "and praying. Dad said to me, 'I pray every day that God sends you a wonderful man to love you and take care of you and Lindsay.'" Two months later, Jane met her future husband, Joe. Dad was able to spend time with Joe, and fourteen months later Jane and Joe were married. It meant so much to my sister that Dad had been able to meet and spend some time getting to know her future husband. She has always felt that Dad had a special hand in their meeting.

By the end of September, Dad was exhausted and so ill that he had to be hospitalized. He was never, ever free of pain, and he developed a terrible case of shingles due to his weakened immune system. This added more excruciating pain and distress to his already-weakened body. We all continued to go home and visit him in the hospital, and my brothers and sisters and I took turns staying during the week. He was never alone; my mother, never leaving his side, stayed with him day and night.

The evening of October 6 my husband and our two daughters returned to visit Dad in the hospital. My poor, poor father—I hated to see him suffering. This was by far the weakest and sickest he had been since Mother's Day. I remember that while riding back to my parents' home that evening, I looked up to heaven and said to God, "He is suffering so. I want him to live, but he is in so much pain. I can't be so selfish in wanting him here for me because of my pain of letting him go. Please God, don't let him suffer anymore."

That evening we convinced my mother, for once, to come home and try to get a good night's rest in her own bed. My sister Kim had never spent the night with Dad in the hospital, and wanted to be with him. My brother Tom, wanting to be close, also stayed with her and my father. Mom hesitated—she almost never spent the night away from him, but tonight she was exhausted. She finally gave in and went home with us to try to sleep.

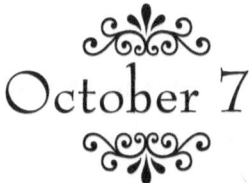

October 7

The next morning, Saturday, was a beautiful fall day. Some of us stopped at a farmer's market on our way back to the hospital to buy apples and treats for the nursing staff. My mother, my husband and I, and some of my other family members went back to the hospital to relieve my sister and brother who had spent the night with my dad. Kim had stayed in the room with Dad and had sat close to him and tried to rest when he did. She told us that Dad had spoken to her, and that he had said, "Get ready, get ready." (Of course at the time she didn't know what he meant, but later realized that Dad knew what was approaching.)

Some of us sat in the room with Dad, and others wandered in and out and sometimes gathered in the small waiting area outside his room. We encouraged our mother and sister to go and get something to eat. I told them that I would sit with Dad while they left for a short while. My mother hesitated; she didn't want to leave Dad. This was a terrible day; he was in so much misery and was so restless. Nothing they were giving him was strong enough to take away his agonizing pain.

We wished there was something we could do for him. We were helpless and it was so very difficult to see him so distressed. Before she left the room, my mother handed me a journal that she and Dad had started to keep months ago, and that she had continued to write in for him. She asked me to write something in it while she was gone. I had no idea what to put down in words, but then I started a letter to my father. I had been holding his hand, and to this day, the only line I remember is the first sentence: "Here I sit Dad, holding your hand. Who's comforting who?"

A nurse came in to check my father and take his vitals. We all left the room and shortly after, there was a lot of commotion. My sister and mother were just returning from their break. We all scrambled to the room along with two other nurses, and we soon knew from the expressions on their faces that my father was dying.

His breathing wasn't normal, and I remember that as I looked at him, I grew weak, feeling dizzy. I started to stagger like I was going to pass out. This time, my sister's boyfriend Joe helped me up and said, "Jody, you have to be strong for your mother." I let him support me, and I tried to compose myself. I moved closer to my father's bed and said, "I love you so much Dad." Everyone kept repeating to him that they loved him and that we would be all right. I heard someone say, "You are the best dad anyone could ever have."

I looked over at my mother and she was dying inside, but she was also trying to be strong for him. She was holding Dad's hands, telling her husband that she loved him so very much and that it was all right for him to let go. Mom told

Dad that she would be all right. She was being courageous, just as she had been for many of the past months. But we knew a part of her was dying along with Dad; he was the only man she had ever loved. Continually, people were saying, "I love you," touching his hands, and just being close to him. We wanted the last words my father heard to be strong and loving, not weak and selfish.

Holding hands, we all surrounded my father and prayed the Lord's Prayer together. The nurses in the room joined us. After a few more breaths, my father was gone.

It is difficult to express, but being with my dear father at his time of death was the saddest, most difficult thing in my life, yet it was so beautiful to be able to comfort and surround him with so much love and peace. We knew that he was not afraid to die, and that he was completely prepared. I thank God that I was there to tell him in his final moments how very much I loved him, and I know he heard me. My father passed away Oct 7, 1989, five months after hearing God's voice.

Answering Our Prayer

We had all prayed for a miracle and we received one on that early morning in May. While receiving the sacrament of the last rites, looking up to God, my father reverently prayed and asked:

"Dear Lord, Please Give Me More Time With My Family."

We witnessed a miracle.

Our father was so close to death, and then God heard and answered his prayer. My father was able to spend private time with each of his children and their families during which he shared his loving and intimate feelings with them. God gave him the strength to travel to each of his childrens' homes, which was something my father was compelled to do. We all felt very blessed with the five extra months we were able to spend together. Our family was able to share in our father's life as he was preparing to meet God, once again.

Our father did not die on May 19 because he had not finished teaching us, loving us, and telling us that we should never, ever be afraid to die. He taught us about faith and trusting in God's will. He had tasks he desired to complete before he went home with his Heavenly Father, and God allowed him more time on earth to attain them. My father accomplished what he felt he needed to do in preparing himself for eternity, and in turn he taught and prepared us. When God spoke to him again on October 7, he went joyfully and peacefully.

My father, Thomas Leroy Strong Sr., is buried
in St. Rose Catholic Cemetery
In Cuba City, Wisconsin. His headstone reads:

Thomas Leroy Strong
July 12, 1923–October 7, 1989

Wife: Geraldine Lois Lightfoot Strong
Children: Jill, Jody, Jane, Thomas Jr.,
Kim and James

And at the bottom it reads:

"WE'LL LOVE YOU FOREVER"

I've **written this true story of my father's last nine months of life not to bring you pain and sadness, but to bring you hope. I wish to help those who are going through a similar situation with a loved one, and those who have already lost someone they love. I believe this will bring and restore faith to all who read this.**

I feel that there was a reason that God chose me to be at my father's bedside the morning that he woke and told me he had "talked to God." My purpose and desire for sharing my father's story with you is to help ease your grief and sorrow. My prayer is that it brings peace to your heart. I want this to encourage and strengthen your belief in God and in eternal life, and to give you confidence that you too will see God and your loved one again, and that they will be waiting for you.

On the morning of May 18, I witnessed a true miracle when my father woke and said to me, "I've talked to God, and I'm to be prepared." God had spoken to him. My father had been near death and he had heard the voice of

God. May 18, 1989 is a day that I will never, ever forget, and a day that I do not want to forget. I am honored that God selected me to hear the words that He spoke to my father.

I know that my father is still with me, and I will always be a part of him. I know that I will see him again; he told me that he would save a spot for me and be waiting.